# Ella's Ear Explorations

## Little Med Minds Series

**Written By:** Christopher Kruglik and Josephine Yalovitser
**Illustrations By**: Josephine Yalovitser

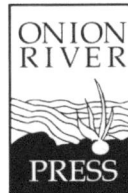

ONION
RIVER
PRESS

Burlington, Vermont

Onion River Press
89 Church Street
Burlington, VT 05401

info@onionriverpress.com
www.onionriverpress.com

ISBN: 978-1-966607-27-4
Library of Congress Control Number: 2025915942

We dedicate this book in memory of Dr. Laurence Coffin, a Vermont heart surgeon and painter whose creativity and accomplishments continue to inspire projects like this one. His legacy lives on through family and friends who carry on his mission to bridge arts and medicine, improving patient education and outcomes through creative and compassionate innovation.

*With heartfelt thanks to Dr. Richard N. Hubbell, whose wise guidance and kind support helped bring this story to life.*

*Little Med Minds* Series: Ella's Ear Explorations

Dive into the world of ear health with **Ella's Ear Explorations**—a magical adventure from the Little Med Minds series! Join Ella as she explores ear tube placement, ear care, and how doctors help keep ears happy and healthy.

*Little Med Minds* is here to:

- Teach kids about their bodies and health in fun and easy ways
- Give kids superpowers like bravery and curiosity, so they can take an active role in their own care
- Answer questions that kids might have about hospitals, check-ups, and more
- Help turn scary moments, like doctor visits or procedures, into exciting learning adventures
- Build trust between children and their doctors
- Spark a love for medicine and science through memorable stories

In this story led by Ella, kids will:

- Learn why some kids need ear tubes and how ear tubes can help
- See how doctors and families team up to keep people healthy
- Better understand the process of having ear tubes placed

**For Parents & Caregivers**:

This book is a tool to start conversations, ease worries, and empower your child. While Ella's journey teaches kids important lessons about their health, always consult your healthcare provider for medical advice.

**Do you love learning with Ella?**

Explore more *Little Med Minds* stories to help grow your child's curiosity and confidence! Available where all books are sold.

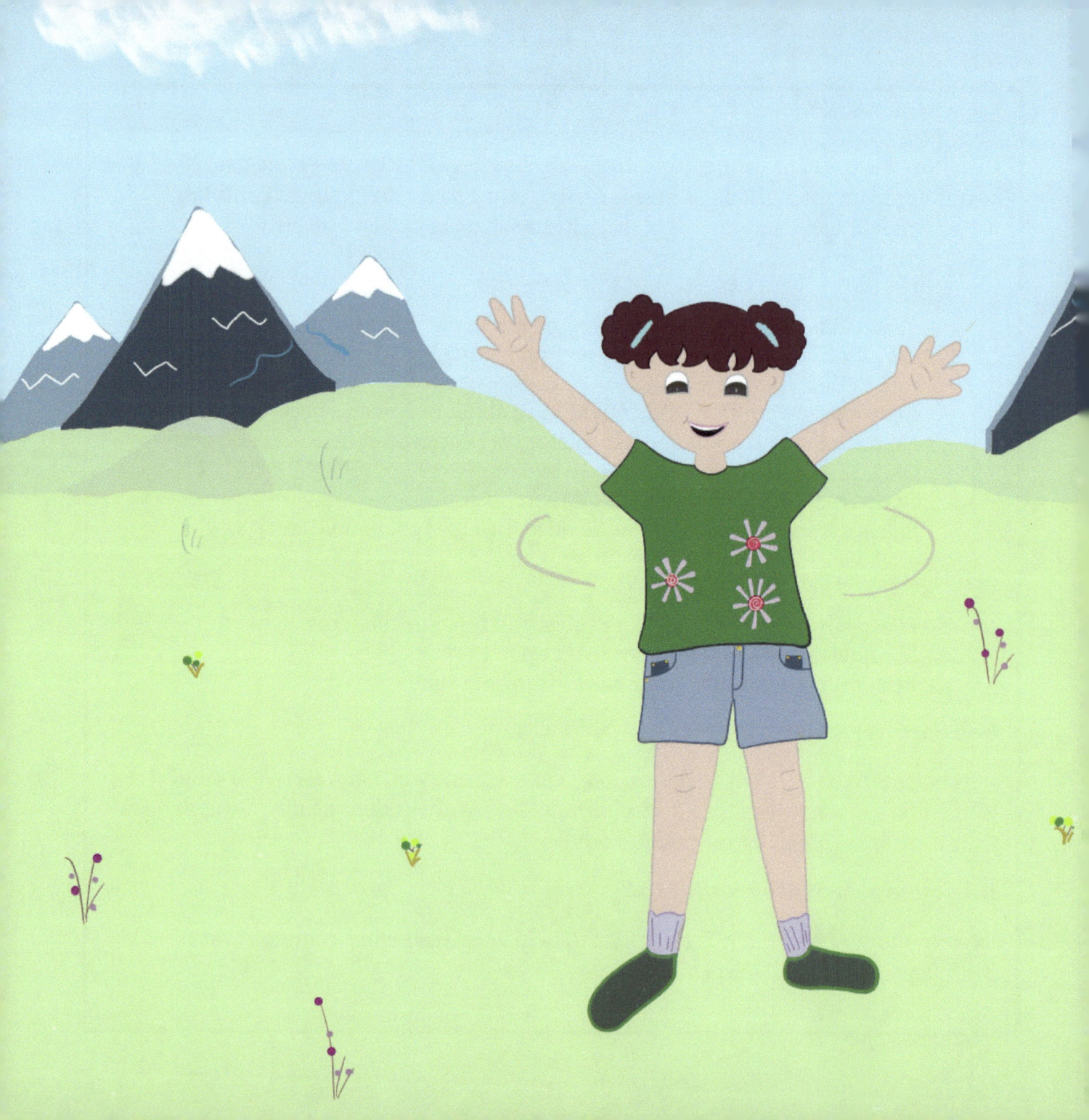

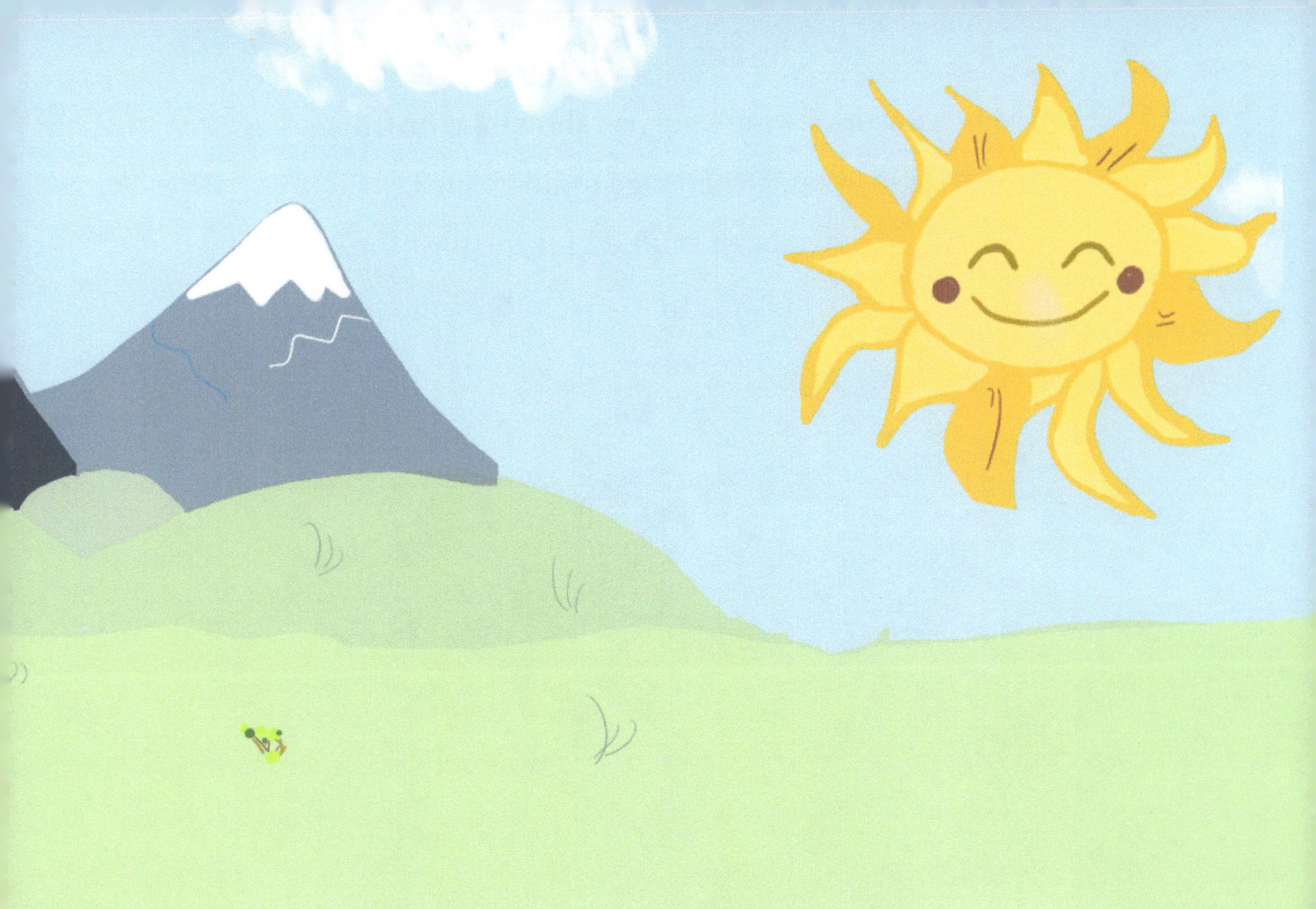

In a nearby village, where the grass was so green
lived a girl named Ella, bright as a sunbeam.
She danced and she twirled, sharing all of her light,
but her ears caused her trouble, all day and all night.

In Ella's world, where giggles should be heard,
ear pain loomed, a challenge quite absurd.
Her hearing had been muffled for the past three months,
she felt icky too often and down in the dumps.

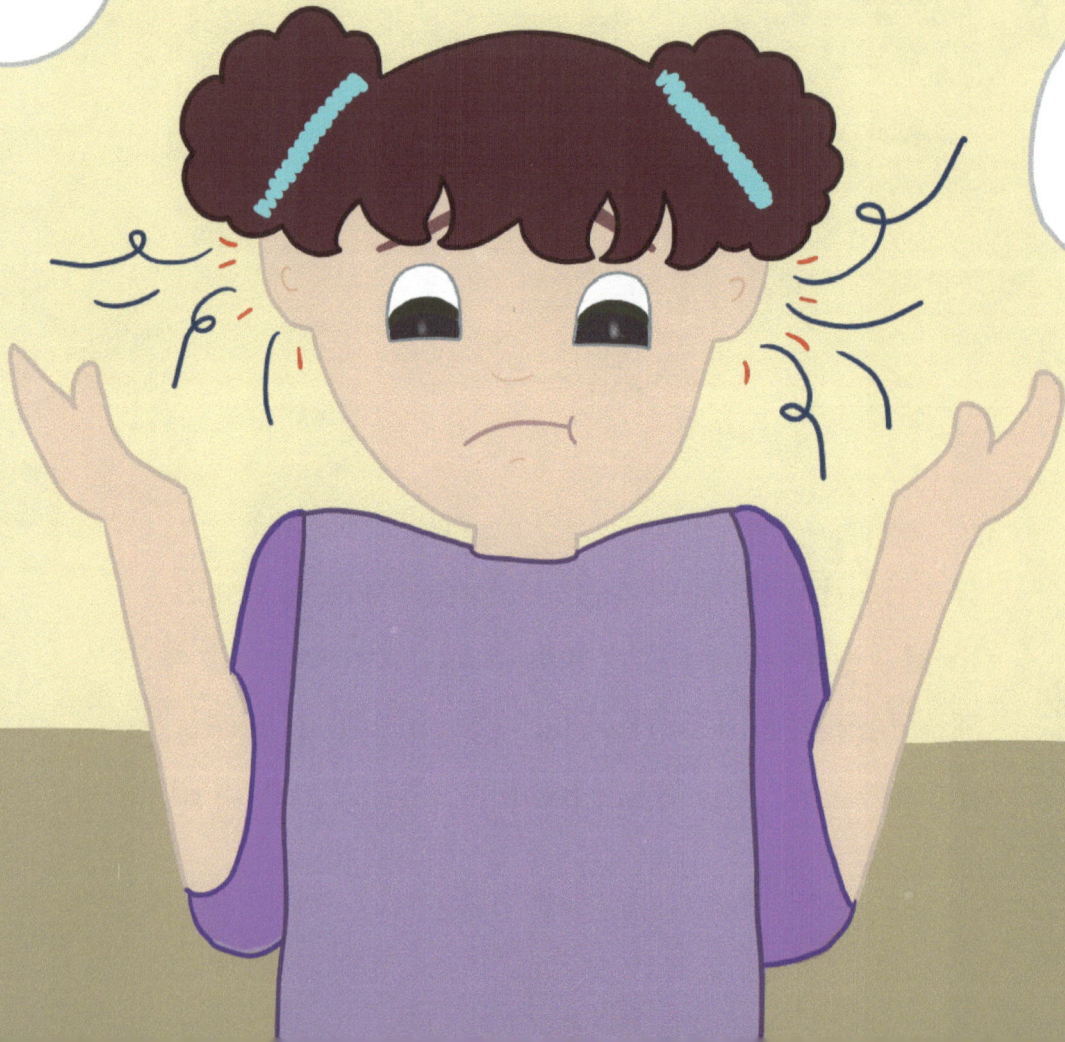

So she hopped in the car with her teddy bear near, and drove off to the doctor to check out her ears.

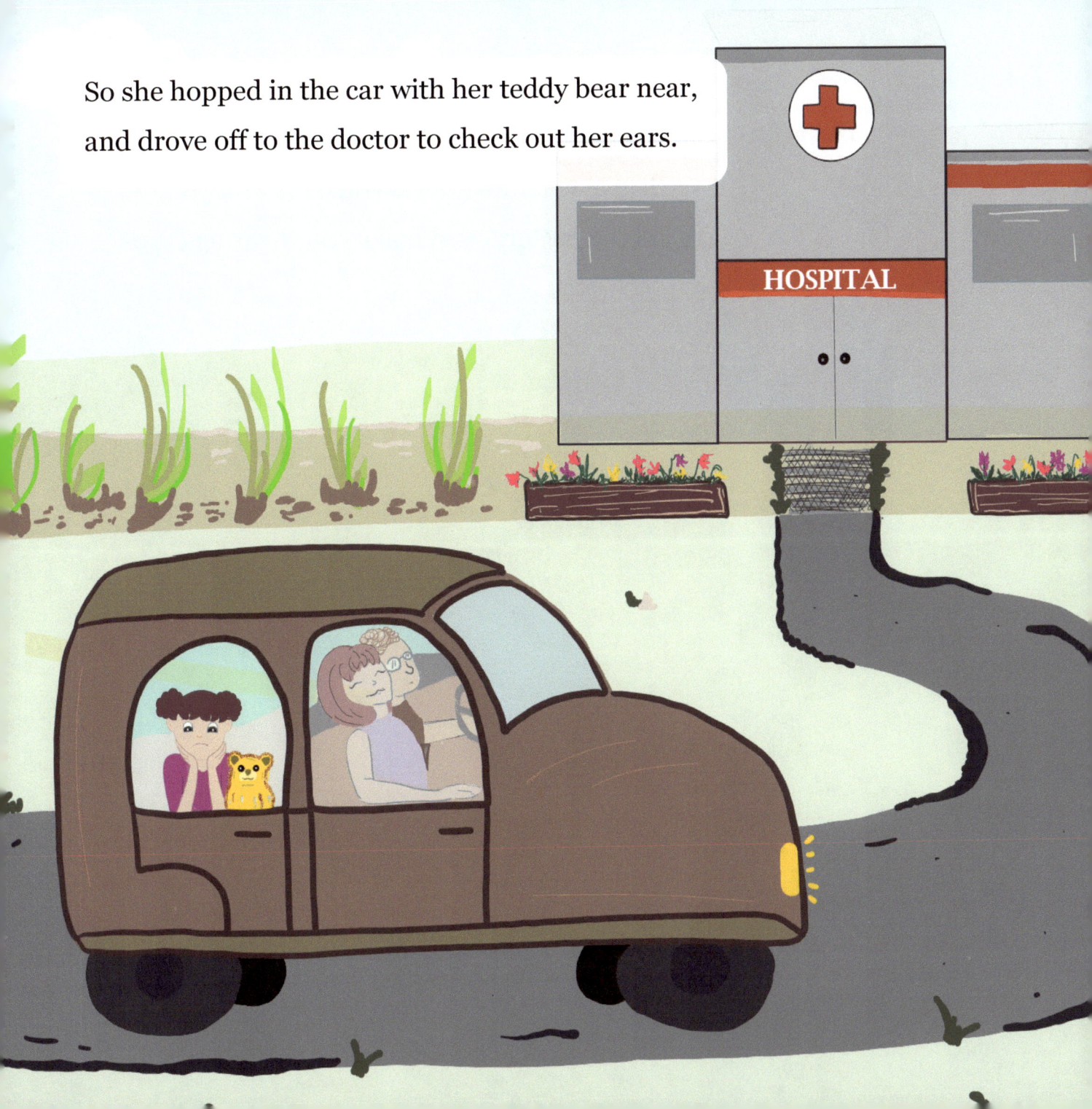

HOSPITAL

The doc smiled widely, with a coat so white, and said, "Ella, my dear, we'll make things alright. We'll give you these meds you'll take for your ear to kill the bacteria and make your hearing clear!"

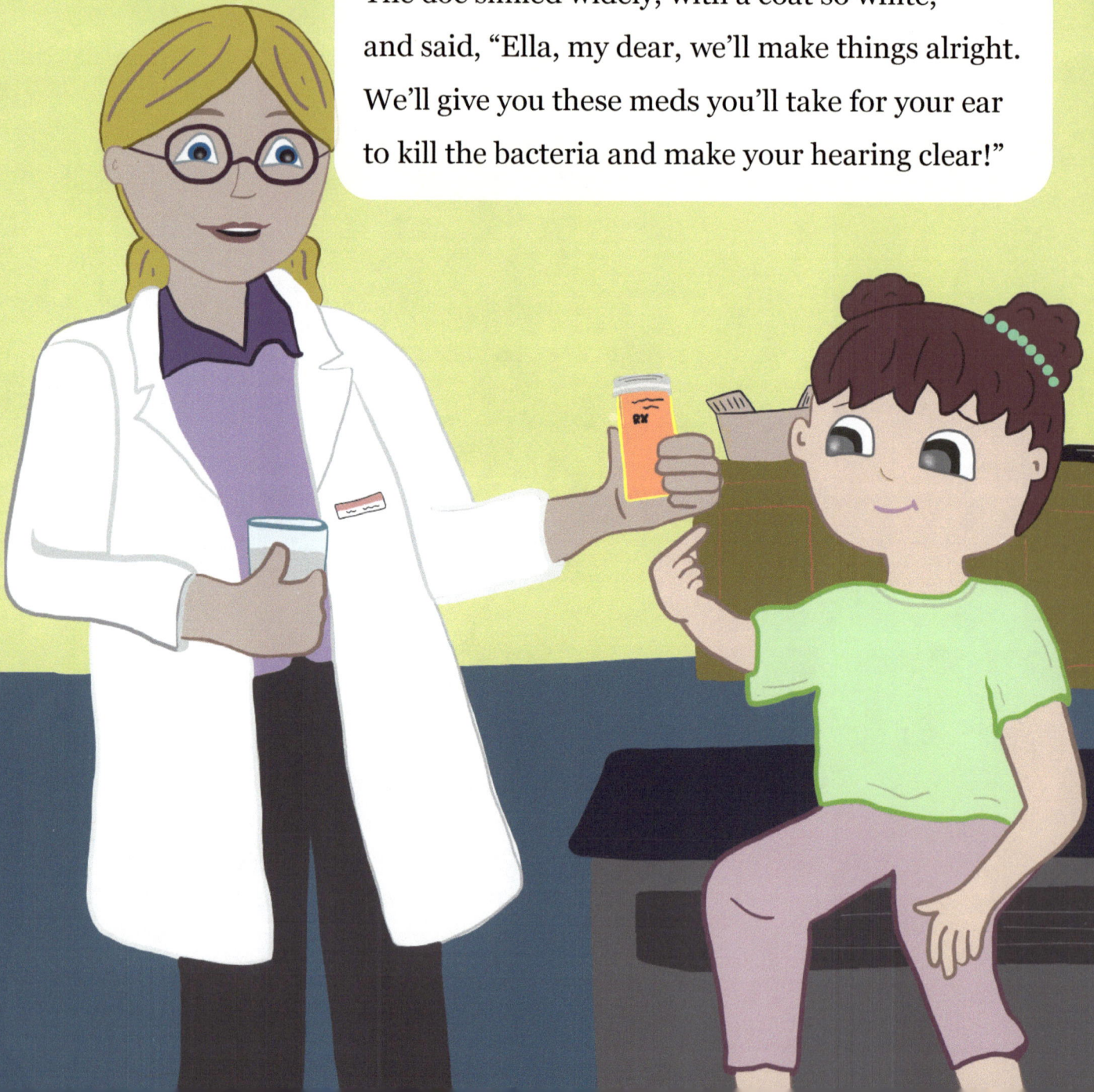

Ella had taken the new medicine all week,

then went to the beach for some fun in the heat.

But she couldn't hear the waves crashing ashore,

and her ears started throbbing and feeling quite sore.

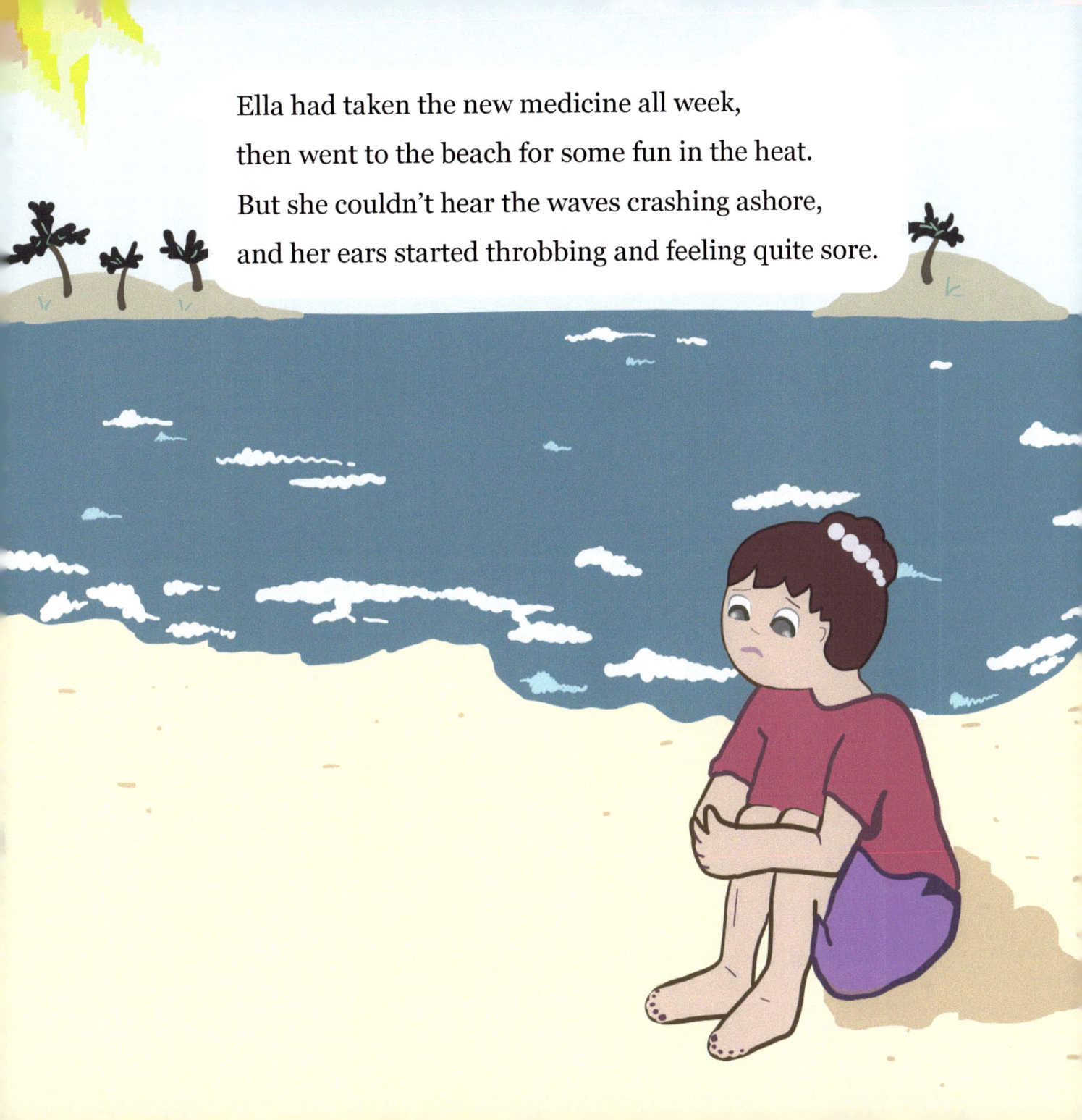

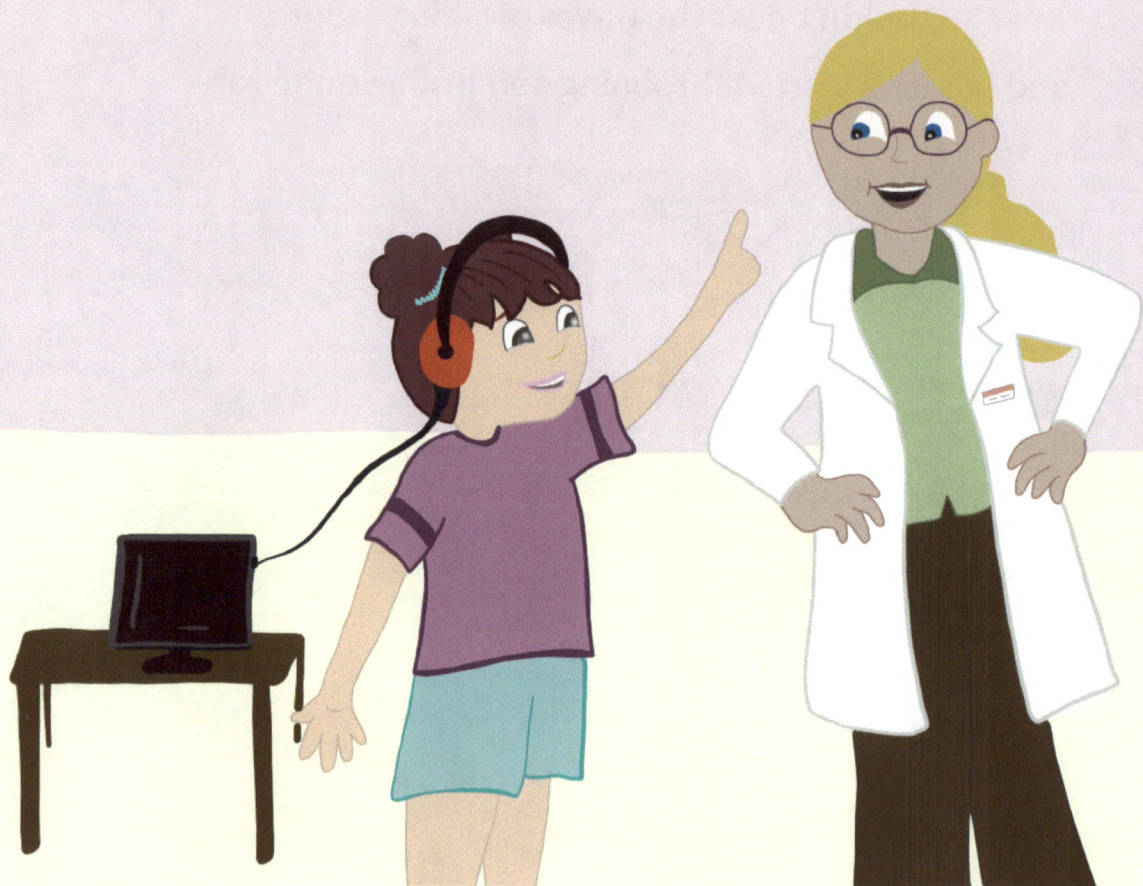

Three times in six months, Ella's symptoms came through,
"The drops aren't helping – we'll try something new.
First thing you'll do is a hearing exam,
You'll listen for a 'beep' and then raise up your hand.

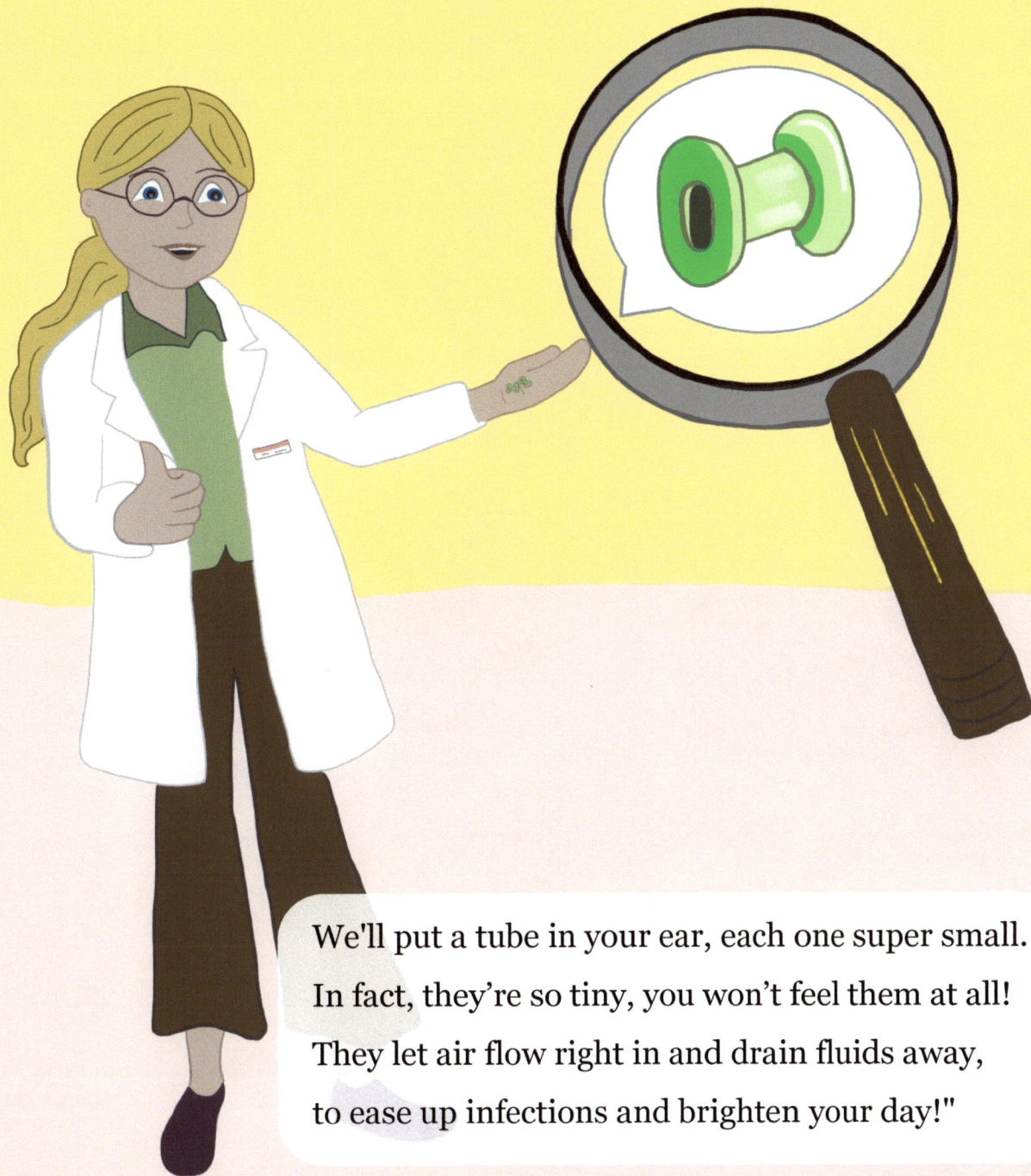

We'll put a tube in your ear, each one super small.
In fact, they're so tiny, you won't feel them at all!
They let air flow right in and drain fluids away,
to ease up infections and brighten your day!"

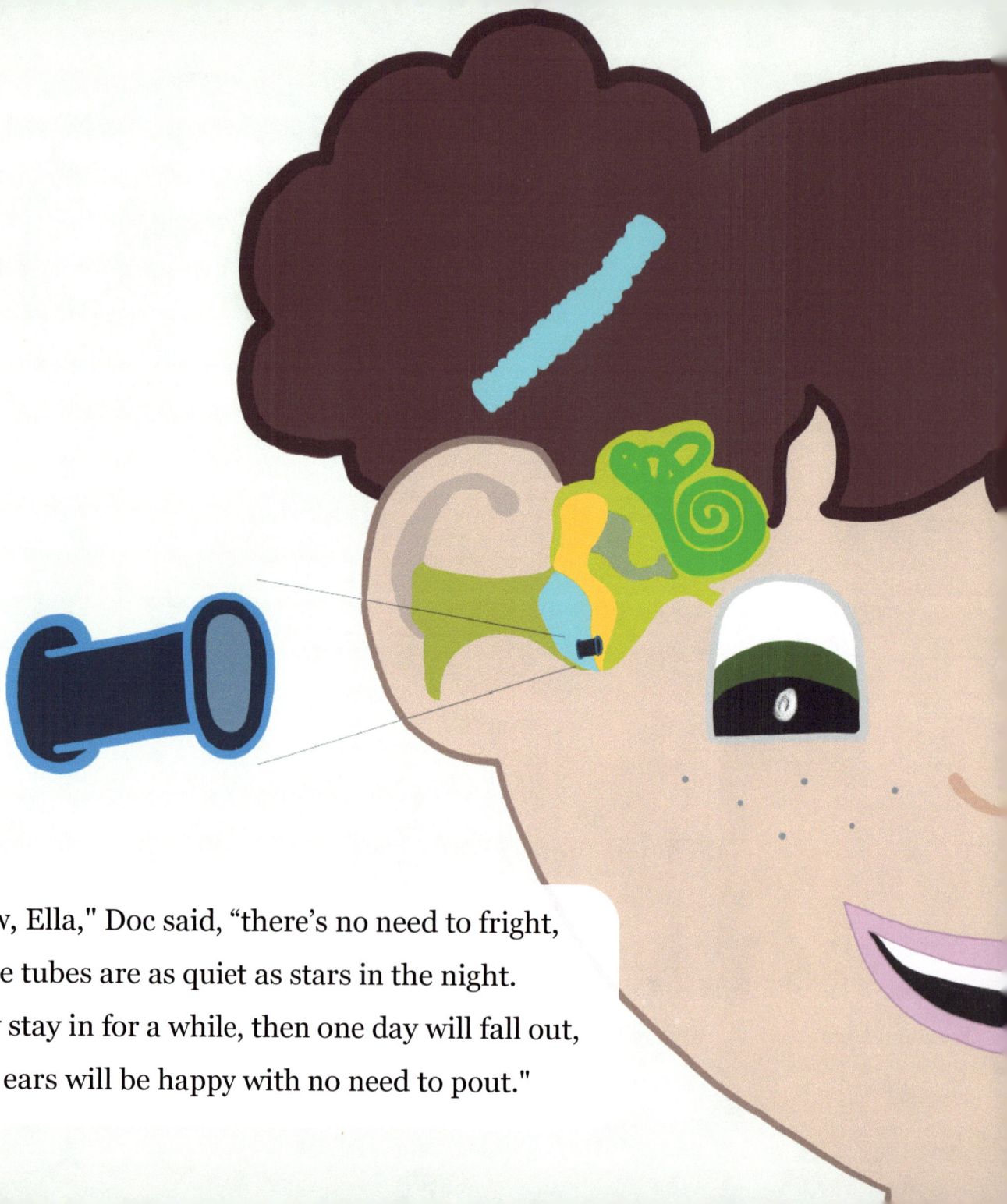

"Now, Ella," Doc said, "there's no need to fright,
These tubes are as quiet as stars in the night.
They stay in for a while, then one day will fall out,
your ears will be happy with no need to pout."

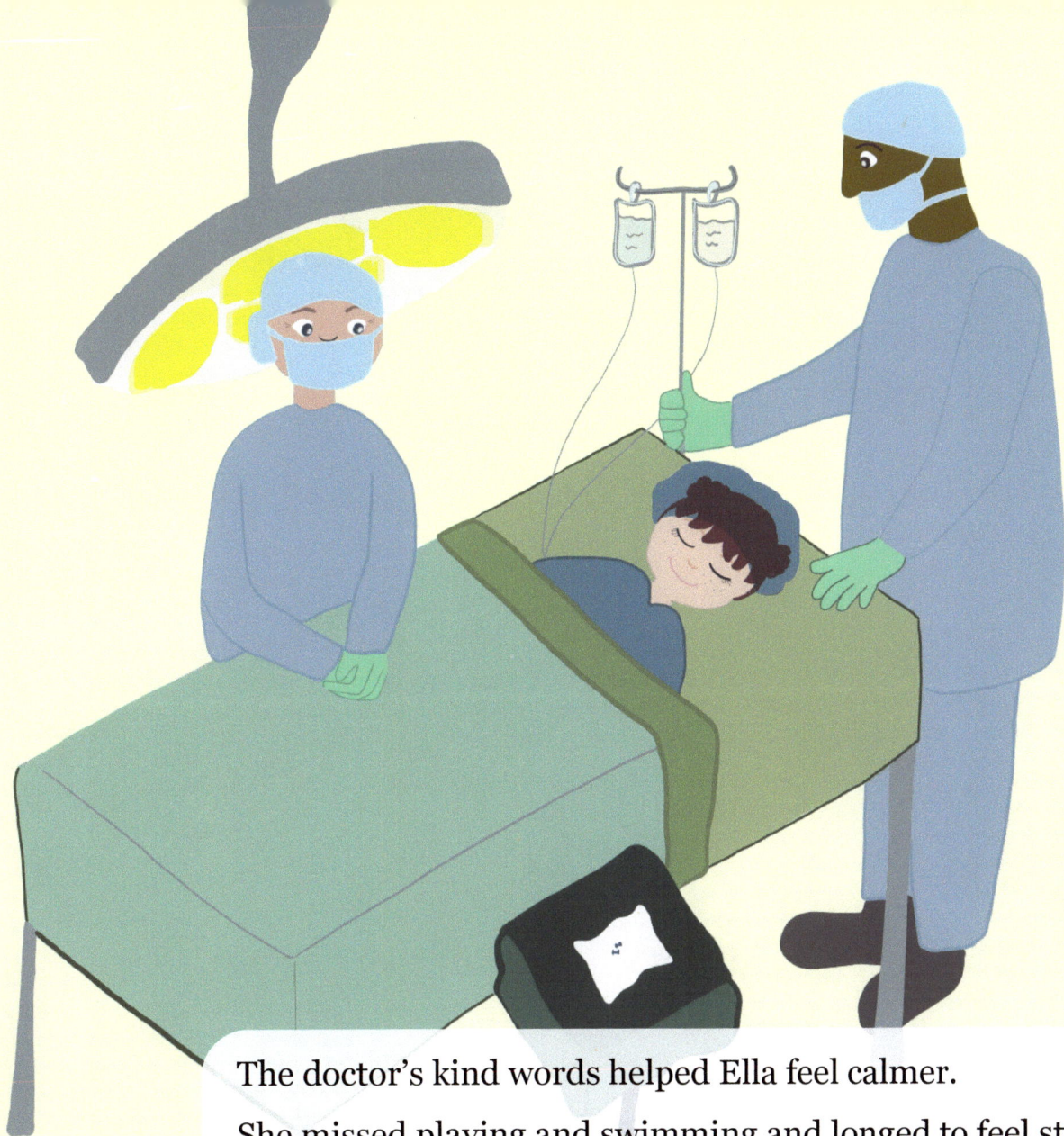

The doctor's kind words helped Ella feel calmer.
She missed playing and swimming and longed to feel stronger.
So bravely she climbed onto the hospital bed,
and fell right asleep with sweet dreams in her head.

She woke up from surgery and said, "That was fast!
I was dreaming of rainbows, but it didn't last."
Her parents scooped her in for a big, warm hug.
And in that very moment, Ella felt so snug.

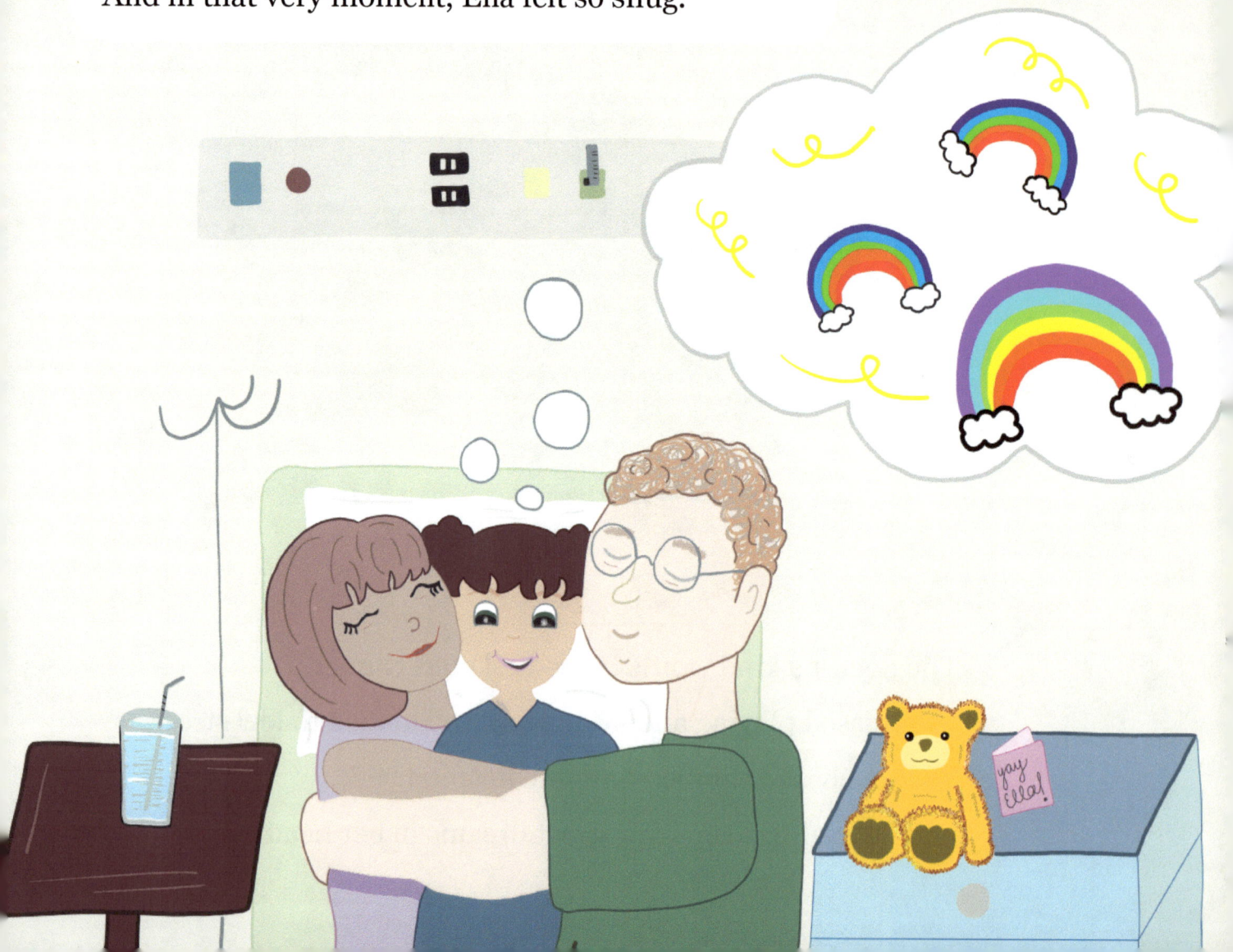

Back home with her friends, Ella listened with glee.
Without any earaches, she was as happy as can be!
At school the next day, everyone sang with cheer,
"Goodbye, ear infections, you're out of here!"

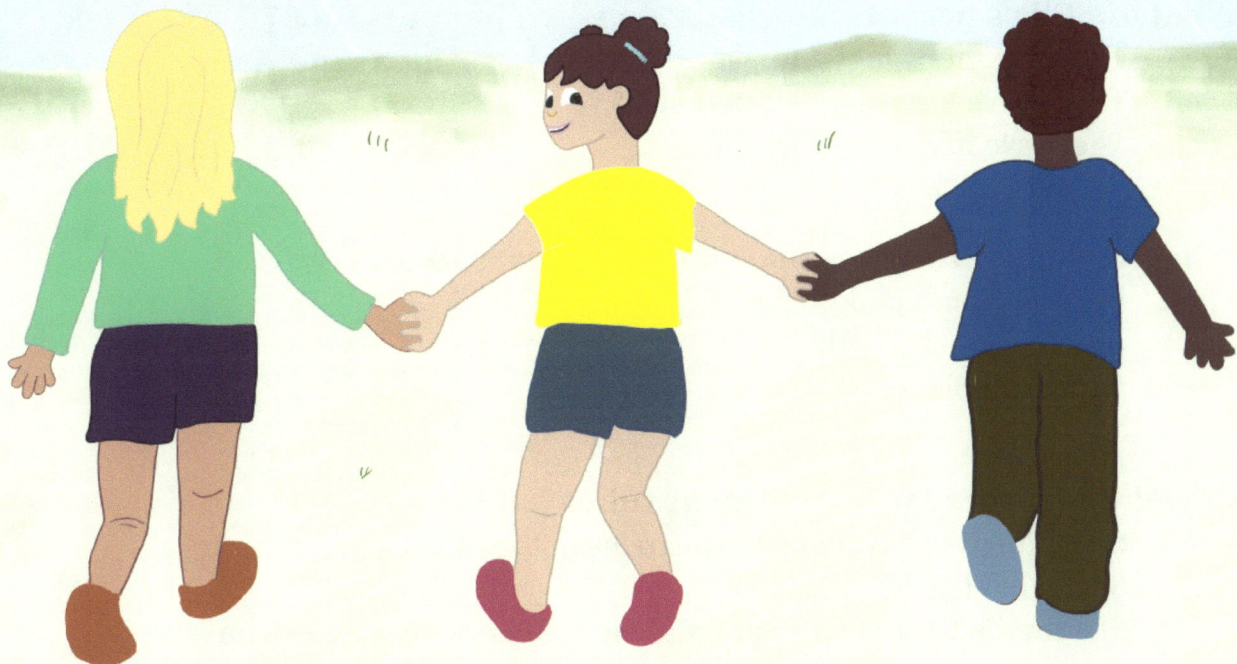

So, friends, if your ears ever feel not so great,
the doctor can help you, so don't hesitate.
Remember dear Ella with ear tubes so small
they brought back her laughter—the best sound of all!

## ELLA'S EAR EXPLORATIONS MINI-QUIZ

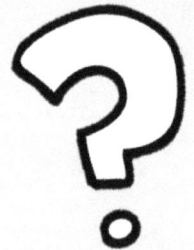

1. **What was causing Ella's ear pain?**
   A. Ear infections
   B. Toothaches
   C. Coughing

2. **What did Ella's parents and sister do when her ears hurt?**
   A. They sang her songs and played outside
   B. They drove her to see her doctor
   C. They gave her yummy ice cream

3. **What were the tiny tubes placed in Ella's ears like?**
   A. Polka dots and pink stripes
   B. As quiet as stars in the night
   C. Rainbow-colored

4. **Why did Ella agree to have the ear tubes put in?**
   A. She wanted to have matching earrings
   B. She didn't like lollipops
   C. She couldn't handle the ear pain and wanted to play and swim

5. **What did Ella's friends say when they saw her at school after the ear tubes were placed?**
   A. "Ella, you're in trouble!"
   B. "Goodbye, ear infections, you're out of here!"
   C. "Let's play video games!"

*Answers: A, B, B, C, B*

# *Meet the Authors*

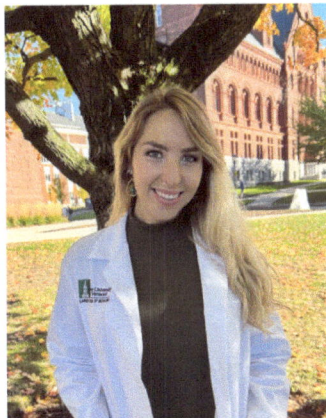

Josephine Yalovitser grew up in Westchester, New York, immersed in Russian culture as the child of immigrants. She discovered her love of the arts early on, with piano and singing at age four. Her work and original compositions have earned national and international recognition, with performances at prestigious venues including Carnegie Hall and Lincoln Center. She went on to study psychology and anthropology at Dartmouth College and will complete her medical degree from the University of Vermont College of Medicine in 2026. Passionate about the intersection of medicine and the arts, Josephine strives to bring creativity, empathy, and a holistic perspective to patient care. Whether through music, medicine, or storytelling, she is committed to healing that honors the full human experience.

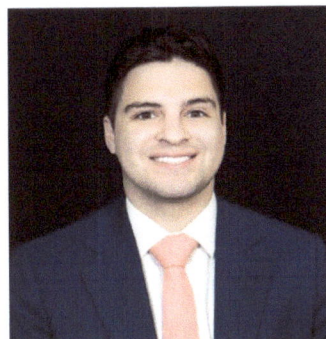

Born in New Haven, Connecticut, in 1997, Christopher Kruglik grew up in the small town of Northford, Connecticut, with his mother and father, two sisters, and two brothers. He went on to receive his Bachelor of Science degree in Biochemistry at the University of Vermont, as well as his Master of Medical Sciences and Master of Public Health. As of 2025, Christopher is currently enrolled in his last year of medical school at the Larner College of Medicine at the University of Vermont. Christopher's clinical interests lie within the sector of the public health realm, pediatrics, and surgery. He is excited to be able to share the *Little Med Minds* book series with his co-author and illustrator to help make children more comfortable and prepared when seeing their physician or getting ready for a surgical procedure.

www.ingramcontent.com/pod-product-compliance
Lightning Source LLC
Chambersburg PA
CBHW061148030426
42335CB00002B/146